COLE ALDERTON

SHE COMES HARD:

Sex guide for men; Make your woman wet at the mere sight of you

Contents

Foreword

Sex. Despite pornography and numerous extremely instructional popular songs,many men still seem pretty clueless about sex.

What compels a lady to lay down with a man? Is it true that a chap can giggle a lady into bed? Does he have to be mysterious or attractive to stand any chance at all?

Sex is evergreen, hot and everything pleasant. There really aren't enough words to describe the exhilarating moment of getting intimate with your partner. At the point when lips and bodies contact, there are firecrackers and blasts that cause you to feel like you're at the highest point of the world. With adoration, trust and grasping come closeness and sex. This extremely intimate act not only gives you and your partner intense pleasure but also helps you with resting soundly, alleviate pressure and deliver cheerful endorphins inside the body.And not to forget, it burns a ton of calories!.

Sex and wellbeing remain inseparable, research has connected it to a slimmer waistline, a stronger heart and a lower risk for prostate and bosom malignant growths. It's likewise a help for psychological well-being,since sex is associated with lower rates of depression and better mood.

Yet, Americans today are having less of it than Americans 10 years ago. Birds do it, bees do it, and men do it any old time. But women will only do it if the candles are scented just right and their partner has done the dishes first. A stereotype, sure, but is it true? Do men really have stronger sex drives than women?

Well, yes, they do. Study after study illustrates that men's sex drives are not only stronger than women's, but much more straightforward. The sources of women's libidos, by contrast, are much more difficult to pin down.

It's common wisdom that women place more value on emotional connection as a spark of sexual desire. But women also appear to be heavily influenced by social and cultural factors as well.

Sexual desire in women is extremely sensitive to environment and con-text,men and women travel slightly different paths to arrive at sexual desire."Some women say that desire originates much more between the ears than between the legs," for women there is a need for a plot;hence the romance novel. It is more about the anticipation, how you get there; it is the longing that is the fuel for desire.

Women's desire is more contextual, more subjective, more layered on a lattice of emotion. Men, by contrast, don't need to have nearly as much imagination, since sex is simpler and more straightforward for them.

Chapter 1

Things Every man Should Know About Sex

Here are 16 things I think all guys need to know about sex

1. **Using sex toys doesn't mean your partner isn't "enough" for you.**

Humans are tool-using primates. We don't think we're inadequate because we use a hammer to build a shelf. Why should we feel inadequate because we use tools to augment our sex play?

Tools make us clever. Sex toys are tools to bring pleasure, fun and maybe a little efficiency to your sex life. What's not to love? Let's have a little less judgment about them and a lot more high-fives about what fabulously clever tool-users we are, OK?

Just make sure they are made from body-safe materials like silicone, stainless steel, glass or hard plastic.

2. **Size matters to some, but not as much as most guys think.**

The average penis is about 5 ½ inches long and that the overwhelming majority of males have penises very near that average.

For most people, this is a huge relief. The only other erect male penises they'd seen were in porn, which are not in any way representative of typical bodies. It'd be like watching the Olympics to get a sense of what you should look like after working out.

What I am saying is that while, yes, size does matter to some people, it doesn't matter to everyone. What is far, far more important is the quality of connection and willingness to co-create a mutually pleasurable experience.

3. **Having meaningful conversations about sex is important.**

I've seen how important it is to bring meaningful conversations about sex into the light.

When we silence these conversations, we create a perfect environment for shame to grow. If we feel shame, we don't seek answers to our most important questions. Misinformation can have consequences, both to our physical and mental Wellbeing.

Sexuality is a big part of most romantic relationships. Being able to communicate about what is and is not working in all aspects of a relationship is key to its sustainability.

When we talk about sex, even with friends, we get better at using the vocabulary. Try saying to a friend, "Hey, I read this interesting article about [insert sex subject here]." Then chat about it. Just align the topic to your level of friendship intimacy and to any previous sex conversations you've had.

When we can create more safe spaces for meaningful conversations about sex, we can help reduce the amount of unnecessary shame around it.

4. **Smokers have weaker boners.**

Lighting up can be a boner killer. Studies show that even occasional smoking in nonsmoking men and women led to reduced genital response. Another interesting study found that male smokers who quit the habit had bigger, firmer erections.

5. Sex just doesn't feel as good when you're sh wasted.

The boner-killing effect it often has in large doses. The fact is, alcohol is a depressant, and you don't want anything dulling your senses when you're having sex.

6. Sex is amazing for your health.

Consider it a naked cure-all…kind of. Research shows it can lower blood pressure and stress, lessen the intensity of migraine headaches, and give your immune system a boost. All good things.

7. Sex burns about three to four calories per MINUTE.

According to a recent study, whereby they measured the calorie expended during sex against actual exercise and found that having sex was about two-thirds of the level of intensity of exercise. And that, is what we call **multitasking**.

8. Orgasms do funny things to your brain.

In those brief seconds of awesomeness, there's a lot going on in your head. *"Parts of the brain associated with reward and pleasure light up, and there's the part associated with fear that tends to shut down."* Recent research also looked at which areas of the brain are involved in which type of stimulation (like clitoral, genital, nipple, etc.). They found that the same areas of the brain light up in response to both nipple and genital stimulation — for both men and women, *so don't skip the nips.*

9. EVERYONE fakes orgasm.

This is true for pretty much everyone, no matter what the gender. Research shows that more than two-thirds of American men and nearly as many women have used lube, and that almost half of the people who reported using lube said that it helps them orgasm. Hey, it's worth a shot!

10. Exercising can get you in the mood.

Research shows that moderate exercise boosts sexual arousal in women, and it can even boost libido in women taking antidepressants. Not to mention, exercise increases your endurance, alertness, strength, and confidence. It gets your blood flowing and boosts testosterone in both men and women. So if you were considering skipping a workout today…maybe don't?

11. **Some people can actually have orgasms from exercise alone.**

"Coregasms" are real, and they're climaxes that can be brought on by ab exercises. About 10% of men and women have reported arousal all the way up to the point of orgasm while exercising. For men, it typically happens during climbing exercises or pull-ups, while women report experiencing it from sit-ups and yoga. It's something about the demand you're placing on your core abdominal muscles.

12. **Oral sex can make a penis get BIGGER.**

A recent study aimed to find out the average penis size by asking men to self-report their erections — and how they got those erections. It turns out the men who received oral before measuring actually reported bigger penises. Of course, these results are only correlational (maybe well-endowed guys were just more likely to ask for an oral favor for the experiment), but it's certainly good to know.

13. **Heterosexual couples secretly wants foreplay to last longer than it does.**

In a study of heterosexual couples, both men and women said foreplay (meaning any kind of sex act that happens before P-in-V sex) would "ideally" last around 18–19 minutes (though women say it realistically lasts about 11 minutes and men say it lasts 13).

14. **Lots of people screw up their birth control, even if they're trying so hard to do it right.**

If you're using condoms plus another highly effective birth control method (like the Pill, the IUD, the ring, etc.), good for you! That means you're protecting yourself against unplanned pregnancy and STDs. A recent study found that about 12% of people did this the last time they had sex…but unfortunately only 59% of them did it correctly. The rest either took the condom off early or put it on after they started having sex. And since many STDs are transmitted via any skin-to-skin contact, that mistake is basically the same as not using a condom at all. So if you're going to double up, do it the right way and keep the rubber on the whole time you're having sex.

15. Most people stop using condoms without talking about STDs and stuff first.

Stop that.

Remember, a lot of STDs are completely symptomless, so just because you love and trust this person doesn't change the fact that they could be harboring something from a previous partner. Do your body a favor and always wear a condom until you're mutually monogamous and have both recently been tested.

16. Talking after sex is a great idea and you should try it!

You know how you sometimes open up like a drunk oversharer after you have sex? That's actually perfectly healthy, especially if you had an orgasm. Recent research shows that people who engaged in pillow talk post-orgasm viewed the talk as more open and intimate, plus they saw greater benefits to opening up to their partners than people who didn't have an orgasm. Blame it on the release of hormones, the warm and fuzzy bonding hormone that's released when you climax.

Importance of sex to women

All women deserve to enjoy a healthy sexual life. pleasure isn't the only benefit of sex. Making love is good for adults, and making love regularly is even better.Studies have shown that sex is extremely beneficial to our health. Sex activates a variety of neurotransmitters that impact not only our brains but several other organs in our bodies.

The benefits of sex for women include:

- Lower blood pressure
- Better immune system
- Better heart health, possibly including lower risk for heart disease
- Improved self-esteem
- Decreased depression and anxiety
- Increased libido
- Immediate, natural pain relief
- Better sleep
- Increased intimacy and closeness to a sexual partner
- Overall stress reduction, both physiologically and emotional

Women, of course, have a variety of different lifestyles, situations, and preferences when it comes to sex. Fortunately, all women can experience benefits of sex, no matter their situation.

Chapter 2

Premature Ejaculation

Premature ejaculation occurs in men when semen leave the body (ejaculate) sooner than wanted during sex. Premature ejaculation is a common sexual complaint. As many as 1 out of 3 people say they have it at some time.

Premature ejaculation isn't cause for concern if it doesn't happen often. But you might be diagnosed with premature ejaculation if you:

- Always or nearly always ejaculate within 1 to 3 minutes of penetration
- Are not able to delay ejaculation during sex all or nearly all the time
- Feel distressed and frustrated, and tend to avoid sexual intimacy as a result

Premature ejaculation is a treatable condition. Medications, counseling and techniques that delay ejaculation can help improve sex for you and your partner.

Symptoms of Premature Ejaculation

The main symptom of premature ejaculation is not being able to delay ejaculation for more than three minutes after penetration. But it might occur in all sexual situations, even during masturbation.

Premature ejaculation can be classified as:
  Lifelong: Lifelong premature ejaculation occurs all or nearly all the time beginning with the first sexual encounter.
  Acquired: Acquired premature ejaculation develops after having previous sexual experiences without problems with ejaculation.
  Many people feel that they have symptoms of premature ejaculation, but the symptoms don't meet the criteria for a diagnosis. It's typical to experience early ejaculation at times.

When to see a doctor
  Talk with your health care provider if you ejaculate sooner than you wish during most sexual encounters. It's common to feel embarrassed about discussing sexual health concerns. But don't let that keep you from talking to your provider. Premature ejaculation is common and treatable.

A conversation with a care provider might help lessen concerns. For example, it might be reassuring to hear that it's typical to experience premature ejaculation from time to time. It may also help to know that the average time from the beginning of intercourse to ejaculation is about five minutes.

Causes of Premature Ejaculation

The exact cause of premature ejaculation isn't known. It was once thought to be only psychological. But health care providers now know that premature ejaculation involves a complex interaction of psychological and biological factors.

Psychological causes

Psychological factors that might play a role include:

- Early sexual experiences
- Sexual abuse
- Poor body image
- Depression
- Worrying about premature ejaculation
- Guilty feelings that can cause you to rush through sex

Other factors that can play a role include:

Erectile dysfunction: Being anxious about getting and keeping an erection might form a pattern of rushing to ejaculate. The pattern can be difficult to change.

Anxiety: It's common for premature ejaculation and anxiety to occur together. The anxiety may be about sexual performance or related to other issues.

Relationship problems: Relationship issues can contribute to premature ejaculation. This may be true if you've had sexual relationships with other partners in which premature ejaculation didn't happen often.

Biological causes

A number of biological factors might contribute to premature ejaculation. They may include:

- Irregular hormone levels
- Irregular levels of brain chemicals
- Swelling and infection of the prostate or urethra
- Inherited traits
- Risk factors

Various factors can increase the risk of premature ejaculation. They may include:

Erectile dysfunction: You might be at increased risk of premature ejaculation if you have trouble getting or keeping an erection. Fear of losing an erection might cause you to hurry through sex. This may happen whether you're aware of it or not.

Stress: Emotional or mental strain in any area of life can play a role in premature ejaculation. Stress can limit the ability to relax and focus during sex.

Complications

Premature ejaculation can cause issues in your personal life. They might include:

Stress and relationship problems: A common complication of premature ejaculation is relationship stress.

Fertility problems: Premature ejaculation can sometimes make it hard for a partner to get pregnant. This may happen if ejaculation doesn't occur in the vagina.

Treatment for Premature Ejaculation

Seeking help for premature ejaculation from a doctor or sex therapist is a good idea. Treatments for premature ejaculation will vary depending on the cause and whether it is lifelong or acquired premature ejaculation. The treatments include:

Behavioural techniques: these include the Semans 'stop-start' technique and the Masters and Johnson 'squeeze' technique

The Semans technique involves learning to control the sensations prior to ejaculation. The idea is to repeatedly bring yourself close to ejaculation, then stop and rest. If you do this often enough, you will learn to recognise your 'point of no return'

The Masters and Johnson technique (named after the famed sex researchers)

involves squeezing the end of the penis just before ejaculation to lessen the urge to ejaculate.These exercises can be done alone or with a partner

Kegel exercises: these exercises are designed to strengthen the pelvic floor. To identify the muscles of your pelvic floor, stop yourself from urinating in midstream. This is the action you need to practice when your bladder is empty. Tightly contract the muscles and hold for 10 seconds. Repeat 10 times, three times a day

psychotherapy and counseling:e of an experienced sex therapist, any underlying anxieties about sex can be explored and eased

reducing penile s**Rs and creams can be used:**o reduce penile sensation and should be applied 30 minutes before sexual intercourse. Use these treatments with a condom to prevent absorption by your partner. Using two condoms may also help to reduce sensation

If premature ejaculation is associated with erectile dysfunction, erectile dysfunction treatments can help restore control of ejaculation.

Chapter 3

The average sex stamina for man in bed

Stamina can mean many things, but when it comes to sex, it often refers to how long you can last in bed.

For males, the average time between the sheets is anywhere from two to five minutes. For females, it's a bit longer: about 20 minutes before reaching the big O.

Things to do to boost your stamina

If you're unsatisfied with how quickly you do the deed, there are a number of things you can try to boost your stamina and improve your overall sexual performance.

1. Masturbation can help build up endurance
   Masturbation can help you last longer in bed by releasing up built-up sexual tension.
   You may find it helpful to:

   • Switch things up by using your non-dominant hand.

- Gyrate and thrust your hips to increase intensity.
- Try different strokes to spice up your solo fun.
- Use one hand to tend to your penis and the other to play with your testicles.
- Stimulate your prostate for a deeper orgasm.

2. Exercise can help build up strength

If you want to increase your stamina, you'll need to build up your strength. A stronger body can endure more, allowing you to last longer between the sheets.

Biceps

Stronger biceps means you can handle more weight when lifting, pulling, tossing, and throwing.

Exercises to try include:

- bicep curls
- chin-ups
- bent-over row

Triceps

Strong triceps not only make pushing easier, but they also build up the power of your upper body.

Exercises to try include:

- bench press
- triceps extension
- triceps pull-down or push-down

Pectoral

You use your pectoral muscles for everything you do; from opening a door to lifting a glass. When you have stronger pecs, you have a stronger body overall.

Exercises to try include:

- bench press
- chest dips
- push-ups

Abdominal

When you have strong abs, you have a more powerful core. And when you have a strong core, you're more balanced and feel less back pain.

Exercises to try include:

- sit-ups
- planks
- high knees

Lower back

A strong lower back stabilizes and supports your spine, as well as helps strengthen your core.

Exercises to try include:

- bridges
- lying lateral leg raise
- superman extension

Pelvic floor

Your pelvic floor controls your genitals, which means if you want to increase your sexual stamina, you need to build strong and flexible pelvic floor muscles.

Exercises to try include:

- Kegels
- squats
- bridges

Glutes

Weak glutes can throw off your balance and stiffen your hips, which will affect your performance in bed.

Exercises to try include:

- squats
- weighted lunges
- hip extension

Quads and hamstrings

Your quad and hamstrings power your hips and knees, which means the stronger those muscles are, the faster and longer you can go.

Exercises to try include:

- leg press
- lunges
- step-up

3. Exercise can also improve flexibility

When your muscles are loose and flexible, you have a fuller range of motion, which means you can do more — a lot more — in bed.

Standing hamstring stretch (for the neck, back, glutes, hamstrings, and calves):

- Stand with your feet hip-width apart, knees bent slightly, and arms resting by your sides.
- Exhale as you bend forward at the hips.
- Lower your head toward the floor, relaxing your head, neck, and shoulders.
- Wrap your arms around your legs, holding the pose for at least 45 seconds.
- Then, bend your knees and roll up.

Reclining bound angle pose (for inner thigh, hips, and groin):

- While lying on your back, bring the soles of your feet together, allowing your knees to open up and move closer to the floor.
- Keep your arms at your sides, palms facing down on the ground.
- Hold the pose for at least 30 seconds.

Lunge with spinal twist (for hip flexors, quads, and back):

- Get into a forward lunge position starting with your left foot.
- Place your right hand on the floor.
- Twist your upper body to the left, extending your left arm toward the ceiling.
- Hold this pose for at least 30 seconds, and then repeat on the right side.

Triceps stretch (for the neck, shoulders, back, and triceps):

- Extend your arms overhead.
- Bend your right elbow, and reach your right hand so that it's touching the top middle of your back.
- Use your left hand to grab just below your right elbow, and pull your right elbow down gently.
- Hold for about 15 to 30 seconds, then repeat with the left arm.

4. Exercise to steady your breath and strengthen your tongue

In addition to relaxing your mind, controlling your breath allows your body to give your muscles more oxygen-rich blood. This can lead to a lower heart rate and may result in a better overall performance.

Strengthening your tongue can also help improve your breathing, as well as increase your stamina for oral sex.

For a strong tongue, try these exercises:

- Tongue pull-back. Stick your tongue out straight, then pull it back in your mouth as far as you can. Hold this position for 2 seconds. Repeat 5 times.
- Tongue push-ups. Push the bottom of the tip of your tongue as hard as you can into the front of the roof of your mouth, right behind your teeth. Repeat 5 to 10 times.

Key nutrients for overall performance

Capsaicin: Capsaicin is found in most hot peppers, so no wonder it helps boosts your endurance. It also speeds up recovery, which means you can go again in no time.

Capsaicin-rich foods include:

- chili peppers
- sweet peppers
- ginger root

Potassium: One of the body's most important electrolytes, potassium keeps your muscles and cells hydrated, aids in recovery, and boosts your metabolism — all of which are important if you want to keep up your stamina.

Potassium-rich foods include:

- banana
- cantaloupe
- spinach
- broccoli
- white potato
- tomatoes
- carrot
- low-fat milk or yogurt
- quinoa

Complex carbs: Simple carbs found in pasta and bread can kill your stamina quickly. But complex carbs do the exact opposite: They help give your body a long-lasting energy boost.

Foods with complex carbs include:

- oatmeal
- yams and sweet potatoes

- whole wheat bread
- brown rice and wild rice
- quinoa, barley, bulgur, and other whole grains
- corn
- peas and dried beans

Protein: Protein takes longer than carbs to break down, giving your body a longer-lasting source of energy.

Foods packed with protein include:

- nuts
- tofu
- eggs
- lean red meat, poultry, and fish
- yogurt, cheese, and milk

B vitamins: B vitamins — especially B-1 to B-5, and B-12 — regulate your sex hormone levels and function, which helps give your libido and performance a boost.

Foods rich in B vitamins include:

- lean meat, fish, and poultry
- eggs
- peanut butter
- avocado
- fortified and enriched grains
- milk and dairy products
- leafy green vegetables

Omega-3s: Omega-3s are essential fatty acids that help balance your sex hormones, giving your libido and stamina a nice boost.

Foods packed with omega-3s include:

- flaxseed, chia seeds, and hemp
- kale and spinach
- walnuts
- mussels
- tuna and other oily fish Specifically for males

L-citrulline: Research has shown that L-citruline, a naturally occurring amino acid, can increase strength and stamina. It also help you maintain an erection.

Foods high in L-citrulline include:

- watermelon
- onions and garlic
- legumes and nuts
- salmon and red meat
- dark chocolate

L-arginine: The body converts L-citrulline to L-arginine, another amino acid that improves blood flow and builds protein.

Foods with L-arginine include:

- red meat, fish, and poultry
- soy

- whole grains
- beans
- milk, yogurt, and other dairy products

Nitrates: Nitrates improves how your muscles use oxygen, which can help enhance your performance — inside and outside the bedroom.

Nitrate-rich foods include:

- arugula, swiss chard, and other leafy greens
- beets and beet juice
- rhubarb
- carrots
- eggplant
- celery

Magnesium: Magnesium is an essential nutrient that plays a key role in everything from energy to brain function. So when your magnesium levels are low, your stamina is depleted.

Foods high in magnesium include:

- whole wheat
- spinach and other dark leafy greens
- quinoa
- almonds, cashews, and peanuts
- black beans
- edamame

Chapter 4

Foreplay

Foreplay matters especially for Women. Whoever said the most important thing in life is to finish strong never had a frank conversation with a woman about the importance of foreplay. When it comes to sexual prelude, men and women don't always see eye to eye. As you prepare yourself for slow, leisurely lovemaking, suddenly your evening turns into an Emeril Lagasse show: Things were cooking, and then … bam! It's over.

It's particularly important for women to have successful foreplay because it takes a woman a longer time [than a man] to get up to the level of arousal needed to orgasm.

A man can just think about sex and have an erection, but for most women, wanting sex is not enough. Foreplay serves a physical and emotional purpose, helping prepare both mind and body for sex. Many women need to be kissed, hugged, and caressed to create lubrication in the vagina, which is important for comfortable intercourse.

Foreplay and the Clitoris

Foreplay also helps the clitoris fulfill its "O" so important role. "It has the same characteristics as the penis,blood flows into the clitoris, and in order for a woman to have an orgasm, there must be lubrication in the vagina, but also the clitoris must get erect." Stimulation is the key to achieving pleasure.

But we're more than just our biology. After all, a girl's got feelings. A woman especially needs emotional assurance that the man she's about to have sex with really wants to be with her. The time and attention given during foreplay can communicate that message in a way the "Wham, bam, thank you, ma'am" approach simply cannot

So,unless you're a member of The Fast and Furious squad, you probably don't go from zero to sixty the second you hop in the car. So why do you think you can go from holding hands to full-on thrusting when you're in the bedroom? Nah, you need some foreplay to ease your way into the main event.

Though you might view foreplay as a seriously delicious appetizer, some foreplay ideas can be the whole damn meal. I mean it: You don't have to make foreplay solely a prelude to intercourse.

In fact, there are many roads to intimacy, and foreplay is one. Foreplay leads us to a deeper sense of who we are and what we prefer sexually.

The more you get in touch with each other's sexual selves (both figuratively and literally), the more comfortable you'll be sharing your desires, fantasies, all that good stuff.

Tips on foreplay

1. Think outside the bedroom.

If your go-to foreplay routine involves a little kissing and touching—then goes right into wham, bam, thank you, ma'am—it's time to mix it up. Foreplay should definitely begin before you get into the bedroom to have sex. Get low-key frisky with your S.O. when you're out to dinner, watching TV in the living room, and anywhere else you're feeling the ~vibe~.

Having fun and doing things that are exciting to each other can be a form of foreplay.

How can something kinda meh lead to oh yeahhh? Well, it's all thanks to (brace yourself for a scientific name) the excitation-transfer theory, which means that when you do a stimulating activity in one domain, the hyped-up feeling you get can then be transferred into another.

So even if you get jazzed flirting over veggies at the farmer's market together (hey, not judging), that's a form of foreplay.

2. Fill your day with foreplay.

After all, who doesn't want breakfast with a side of arousal? Foreplay can start in the morning and can go All. Day. Long. through sexy little suggestions here and there. Maybe you hop in the shower with them before work (save the shower sex for the main event) or text them a sexy little something during their lunch break (more on that in a sec).

Whatever you're into, you can have lots of moments of foreplay leading up to sex that happens later. In fact, just knowing you're not going to get it on until later that night or even the next day can ramp up the anticipation and make foreplay feel even hotter.

3. Sext them sultry little somethings.

Sexting can be a hot form of foreplay, especially when it includes teasing the person on the other side of the screen. Let your partner know what you're going to do to them when you see them, or hint at what you'd like them to do to you.

Something like "It was so great the last time we _____. I loved it when you touched me in this way, or when you sucked on that." You can head down the sweet and sensual route or go straight-up pornographic. If it feels right in that moment, you can't go wrong. Anything that creates anticipation and arousal is great.

4. Send a sexy pic.

Sure, dirty talk is hot, but a picture leaves a lot less to the imagination. Assuming your partner is someone you know and trust (important detail!), why not send a little something to start setting the mood before they even get home?

5. Spell it o-u-t.

When you're flirting or sexting with your partner, let them know exactly what you find attractive about them. Even if you think they already know because of the whole wanting-to-have-sex-with-them thing, it never hurts to remind them how much their abs, ass, or even ambition turns you on.

"The language of sex is a lot different than the language you commonly use in your relationship vocabulary,you can be going through your day and communicating back and forth in very respectful, egalitarian ways, but you may also jump into some language that's very erotic or sexual."

Basically, whenever the opportunity to seduce your partner presents itself, seize it. And when it doesn't…create it.

6. Play up the sexiness of not being able to have sex (yet).

Crank your next date night up a notch—or ten—by teasing your partner when you're cuddled up at a cozy restaurant or low-lit bar. Teasing is really important because when we can't have what it is that we want, that creates desire.

Whisper in your partner's ear about what you're looking forward to that night, nibbling on their neck, or discreetly touching them wherever they'll take notice. When you know you can't have sex, it becomes all the more arousing.

7. Use psychological lube.

The last thing you want to think about when getting frisky is your errand list or a work project. To simply put, not being in the right headspace can be enough to kill your boner.

That's why it's important to add "psychological excitement" into your foreplay routine, rather than relying solely on physical touch and stimulation.

But what qualifies as psychological excitement? Turns out, tons of sexy stuff: listening to an erotic podcast, watching porn together (there's audible porn now, too), reading erotica aloud to each other, and even playing sex games.

8. Watch each other undress

With sex, we often go on autopilot, and we forget to take in every moment, especially if you've been together for a long time. Instead, make a note to actually watch each other undress. Don't touch each other while it's happening either; make it all about the experience of looking at each other and getting excited just at the thought of how hot you both are.

9. Talk dirty

Instead of actually touching each other, simply tell each other what you want to do. Don't be afraid to go into detail! To make it extra sexy, don't wait until you're in the bedroom. Simply talking about all the dirty, sexy, crazy things you want to do to each other while you're sitting on the couch keeps things fun and flirty.

10. Listen to music

If you don't already turn up your speakers while you're having sex, now might be the time to start. Whatever kind of music turns you both on, whether it's R&B, country, slow songs, or even show tunes, turn it up and use the music as the rhythm of all of your moves. Dance around the kitchen and sing along. Having fun together is sexy! Making a playlist together of your favorite songs to get down to can also be a form of foreplay on its own.

11. Play with ice

Ice is quite possibly the highest ROI on any sex toy. It's entirely free and has benefits for both partners. It's a different and unique sensation to play with temperature during sex. Some ideas for adding ice into your foreplay includes in your mouth during kissing, in your mouth during oral sex, rubbing it down your partner's body, or on you or your partner's nipples. If ice is too much for you and you don't mind getting a little messy, dripping ice cream down your partner's body (or yours!) can do the trick (and it tastes freaking good!). Be careful of using any foods near the vagina in the penis to avoid infections.

12. Go somewhere that reminds you of your relationship

Go back to your first date spot, where you got engaged, where you said "I love you" for the first time, and more. Being in those special places again can bring you back, mentally and physically, to earlier parts of your relationship. It'll remind you how far you've come as a couple … and if that isn't just a little sexy to you, I don't know what is.

13. Make a bucket list together

Sitting down together to come up with everything you want to do this year sexually is the perfect foreplay for the adventurous couple. The items can be as crazy or as tame as you want them (we recommend ideas like having a threesome, talking about sex more, using sex toys, and having multiple orgasms!). Keep this list somewhere where you can go back to it, such as your nightstand, and make it a goal to do one new thing every week. You won't even know how to choose what to do first!

14. Take a shower together

While your partner's in the shower, feel free to hop in! Shower sex doesn't have to be the end goal of this either. Having fun in the water and getting excited for whatever's to happen outside of the shower is exciting all in itself. However, am not against trying to make shower sex work — just don't hurt yourself!

Chapter 5

Sex Positions

While porn may have you think you need to be hung like a horse or need to plow like a jackhammer in order for your partner to reach climax, that is far from the truth. A lot of what you want to focus on is external (the clitoris) and within the first few inches of the vaginal canal.

The first third of the vaginal canal is most pleasure-prone as it is enmeshed in the clitoral structures, so interspersing slow shallow strokes with deeper strokes are bound for their pleasure.

Additionally, some pressure against the cervix also lights up the somatosensory cortex in the brain, along with clitoral and nipple stimulation.

This means an ideal sex position to help your partner orgasm would include clitoral consistency, breast stimulation, and intermittent cervical contact. In simpler terms, make sure you can stimulate her clitoris (using your fingers or a sex toy works too), have access to caress their breasts and pinch their nipples, and lastly, throw in some deep strokes as well.

Different Sex Positions You Have To Try

1. All Access sex position

How it works: Kneel and straddle her left leg while she's lying on her left side. From here, she should bend her right leg around the right side of your waist—allowing full access to her vagina.

This position is an upgrade from standard missionary because this sets you up for deeper penetration and allows you to slow your roll.

With your partner on her side, the girth of your penis will be hitting and emphasizing her g-spot in unique ways, while also allowing you to maintain a clitoral connection, which is often sacrificed in positions that emphasize g-spot stimulation.

Spend some time exploring her body. This setup gives you complete access to her clitoris for manual stimulation. But don't feel limited to solely hands-on fun.

Try withdrawing your penis and, while holding the shaft with your left hand, rub the head against her clitoris. Start out soft and slow, then as you increase speed and pressure, reinsert once you've brought her to the brink of an orgasm.

2. Stand and Deliver sex position

How it works: Stand at the edge of a bed while your partner lies back and raises her legs to her chest. Her knees are bent as if she's doing a "bicycling" exercise. Grab her ankles and enter her. You'll want to start by thrusting slowly, as the deep penetration may be initially painful.

For heightened pleasure have her place her heels on your shoulders, which will open her hips so her labia press against you. This position is also great for manual clitoral stimulation.

3. Spooning sex position

How it works: You both lie on your sides facing the same direction with you behind your partner. She bends her knees and pushes her rear back toward you for easier access to her vagina. Adjusting the lean of your bodies will vary the angle of entry and help with rocking and thrusting.

For heightened pleasure; From here you can reach around and play with her breasts. Depending on the angle, you can potentially stimulate her clitoris manually. This position allows for deep penetration and body contact.

4. Legs on Shoulders sex position

How it works: While she's on her back, have her drape her legs on your shoulders. The angle of her body should be roughly 90 degrees.

This legs on shoulders move should be considered a staple, as it allows for deep vaginal penetration. If the standard G-Whiz isn't doing anything for her, try grabbing her butt and tilting her pelvis upward, slightly toward you. As always, ask her what feels best; a small tweak can be the difference between her not orgasming and orgasming within minutes.

It's a great position for both clitoral and cervical stimulation as well as eye-to-eye lovemaking and attunement.

For heightened pleasure, wrap your arms behind her neck and upper back, lifting her up gently. This not only helps her receive deeper penetration, but also feels more intense, since it forces you both to look into each other's eyes.

5. Cowgirl sex position

How it works: You're lying down on your back. She straddles you with one leg on each side of your torso.

There are numerous variations to cowgirl, and it's worth figuring out with your partner which one works best for her. She may prefer to have her feet planted on both sides of you, so she's squatting on you as opposed to downright riding. She may like it when she leans back because it allows for deeper penetration. She may like when you do all the thrusting—but typically, what facilitates quicker orgasms is when she's in control. She's the one setting the pace, how deeply you penetrate, and which angles you hit. When she's in control, she can give herself everything she needs to orgasm.

It's also great for guys who come first, as you can still grind your penis against your partner as you're losing your tumescence (erection).

6. Happy Baby Pose sex position

How it works: she lies on her back with her legs bent and up in the air. Her legs are slightly past shoulder-length apart, and she's gripping the soles of her feet with her hands.

If your partner is a yogi, she's going to appreciate bringing her yoga practice into the bedroom. And even if she's not into yoga, she'll appreciate the orgasm you help give her. Happy Baby Pose allows you to hit all her angles while she's on her back. It's also an ideal position if you want to engage her clitoris too. With one hand you can stimulate her clitoris, and with your other free hand, you can hold onto her for support.

Happy Baby Pose is also an ideal position for anal sex, during which you can digitally penetrate their vagina and/or play with their clitoris.

7. Child's Pose sex position

How it works: She sits on her heels and then lean forward. While remaining on her haunches, she extends her hands forward; all the while, her back remains straight.

If she has a bad back, this position is great since it elongates her back muscles. Even if she don't have back pain, this position is really relaxing. That's why it's often the neutral pose during yoga, when you need a break from doing other, more strenuous poses.

When they're relaxed during sex, they're more likely to have an orgasm. That's not to say you can't go hard in this position, you can and should if that's what they like, but this position is ideal for both relaxation and deep penetration.

For heightened pleasure, have her grip the bed frame for stability, so you can penetrate harder and deeper.

8. The Standing Dragon sex position

How it works: Position her on the edge of the bed, posing on all fours. As you stand behind her, have her arch her back so it lifts her butt upward.

With your legs outside of hers, use your thighs to squeeze her knees together, which tightens her vagina around your penis. It's the squeeze of the knees together that will provide pleasurable friction against your penis and stimulation of the vestibular bulbs that are part of the clitoris and press against the vagina at the entrance. This position is ideal for G-spot stimulation and also gives you a great view of her curves.

9. Flatiron sex position

How it works: Have her lie face down on the bed with her knees slightly bent and hips slightly raised. For comfort, and to increase the angle of her hips, you can suggest placing a pillow under her lower abs.

From here, enter her from behind and keep your weight off of her by propping yourself up with your arms. This position creates a snug fit—which intensifies her pleasure by making you feel larger to her. This is a great position for increasing your friction, achieving full penetration, while also stimulating her G-spot.

You'll last longer in this position if you switch to shallower thrusts and deeper breaths.

10. Double the Pleasure sex position

How it works: Lie on your back and bend one of your legs, keeping the other outstretched. Have her straddle the raised leg with a thigh on either side and then lower herself onto your member so that her back is facing you.

From here, she should hold your knee and use it for support as she rock up and down.

This position is great because it's a lot like the reverse cowgirl, but with a twist. Raising your knee allows her to rub against your thigh—which produces optimal clitoral stimulation.

Chapter 6

Tantric Sex

Tantric sex is a slow, meditative form of sex where the end goal is not orgasm but enjoying the sexual journey and sensations of the body. It aims to move sexual energy throughout the body for healing, transformation, and enlightenment.

Proponents of tantric sex believe that tantric techniques may help resolve sexual complications such as premature ejaculation, erectile dysfunction, or anorgasmia.

Knowing one's body

Tantric sex encourages people to get to know their own bodies and become in tune with them. By understanding the desire of one's own body, one can incorporate this during sex with a partner. This may lead to greater sexual fulfillment and more intense orgasms.

To understand what one's body wants, it can be useful to engage in tantric self-love or masturbation.

If a person finds that they have emotional blocks around self-touch, they should be curious and gentle with themselves as they explore what is preventing them from getting to know their own body more intimately. The more a person knows about their body and pleasure zones, the more likely they are to have a satisfying sexual experience.

If someone does not wish to engage in masturbation and has a partner, however, they may feel more comfortable learning about their own body through partnered sex.

Knowing one's partner's body

Tantric sex is about honoring one's body and the body of one's partner. By taking time to get to know one's own body as well as that of one's partner, it can help make the experience fulfilling for both people.

A person may consider giving their partner a slow, full-body massage to learn about their body and help awaken their sexual energy. This may also help a person become in tune with their partner's wants and desires.

As is the case with any sexual activity, if at any point a person or their partner becomes uncomfortable, the activity should stop.

How to prepare For Tantric Sex

There are a few things a person or couple can do to help prepare for tantric sex. For example, they can:

- **Prepare the mind:** Focusing on the moment can be difficult if a person is experiencing stress or has many things on their mind. Meditating or stretching before tantric sex may help achieve a clear mindset.
- **Find a good place:** Environment has a key role in tantric sex. Ideally, it will take place in a relaxing setting with a comfortable temperature. A person may want to dim the lights, light a scented candle, or put on

relaxing music.

Building the moment with oneself

To build the moment with oneself, a person can try the following tips:

- **Practice mindfulness:** Tantric sex encourages people to be present in the moment. A person should focus on their breathing and bodily sensations.
- **Explore the body:** Giving a self-massage in which the person pays attention to their touch and body may help heighten physical sensations and arousal.
- **Masturbate:** A person may wish to engage in tantric self-love. Like with partnered sex, the goal of this may not be orgasm. Instead, people may do this to try to feel more connected with their own bodies.

Building the moment with a partner

To build the moment with a partner, people can try the following tips:

- **Adopt a hand-on-heart position:** To gain a deep connection, couples should sit cross-legged and face each other. Both partners should place their right hand on the other's heart, with the left hand atop their partner's. Feel the connection and try to synchronize breathing.
- **Do not go linear:** Normally, sexual activities might follow a script of foreplay, intercourse, and orgasm. However, tantric sex is about experimenting, so it is best to stay open to what feels good in the moment.

- **Make eye contact:** Making eye contact may help deepen the connection and heighten intimacy.
- **Take things slow:** Tantric sex is meditative and about exploring sensations in the moment. This process should be a slow and enjoyable journey for both partners.

Breathing technique

Breathing is an integral part of tantric sex. This is partly because tantric sex revolves around meditation.

During tantric sex, a person should focus on breathing deeply through the diaphragm. To achieve this, they should take a deep breath through the nose for five counts. They should feel their stomach inflate. They should then exhale through the mouth for five counts.

When engaging in tantric sex with a partner, synchronizing the breath may increase connection and intimacy.

Positions In Tantric Sex

There are many positions that people can try during tantric sex.

1. Yab-yum

In Yab-yum, you sit with your legs crossed, and your partner sits on your lap, wrapping her legs around your waist.

You both then embrace and attempt to synchronize your breaths. If you both want to, you can rub your genitals against each other, engage in penetrative sex, or just sit there in the moment.

This position is also suitable for masturbation. A person can sit cross-legged with their back straight, place their palms on their knees, and begin deep breathing.

A person may wish to try this in front of a mirror to learn more about their body.

2. The relaxed arch

For this position, one partner sits on the bed or floor with their legs straight. The other partner then gets on their knees and sits on their partner's lap. The partner on top then slowly leans back and rests their head between their partner's legs.

Tips To Enjoy Tantric Sex

Some tips to better enjoy the experience of tantric sex may include:

1. Explore and experiment

Tantric sex may be a completely new experience for some people. It is useful to engage in self-exploration by oneself or with a partner.

It may also be useful to experiment with the different aspects of tantric sex to find what works for oneself and one's partner.

2. Be comfortable

There is no need to be naked during tantric sex, and most positions are possible with and without clothes.

It is up to the couple whether they wish to start naked, start with clothes on and then get naked, or keep their clothes on throughout the experience.

3. Use the senses

Tantric sex encourages the use of all five senses. By being mindful and in the moment, people can focus on all the senses they are experiencing in the sexual encounter. This can enhance the experience.

Tips To Remember

Tantric sex is a meditative sexual practice that encourages people to focus on mind-body connections. This can lead to fulfilling sexual experiences and greater intimacy.

When preparing for tantric sex alone or with a partner, it is good to set aside some time and find a comfortable environment. This can help people focus fully on the experience.

Breathing is a key component of tantric sex, as it helps a person focus their mind and be in tune with one's body. Tantric sex with a partner encourages the synchronization of breathing to promote connection and intimacy.

Chapter 7

Sex Toys

Some of the unenlightened see vibrators and dildos as replacements for a partner. But a sex toy is only an enhancement. Toys are an appetizer; your partner is the main course.

Seriously, how often are you completely satisfied by an appetizer? Sex toys are designed primarily to get you warmed up, and it's common knowledge that women typically need more to warm up than men.

If you embrace sex toys, you may just find out they make your job easier. Integrating a quiet vibrator into your lovemaking can make her extra-happy.

Guys, the unfortunate reality is that nearly all penises are wired the same. They're fairly easy to figure out and are pretty much idiot-proof. Most women could meet a stranger and have relatively little trouble figuring out how to give him an orgasm.

Women (and their mysterious genitalia) are a whole different animal. Some women can orgasm in 30 seconds, but some take five minutes, and some take 40 minutes or more. Even worse? The sad fact is that some women can't get off at all.

If it takes your woman 40 minutes or more to reach orgasm, why not add in a toy that could make it easier for both of you? That's when you need sex toys that will help make your woman orgasm. With a small vibrator, you can use the soft vibration on her nipples, her neck, and her back — her entire body, really. Move it around slowly on her lower tummy, or try using a little more pressure with it on her pelvic bone.

Take the toy and tease her a bit with it to get her warmed up. But don't just plunge right in. Make sure she's warmed up and lubricated before you allow it to touch her clitoris. If she isn't lubricating on her own, don't take that as a personal affront to your skills. Sometimes it's hormonal and sometimes it's just how we're wired.

If you take the time to help the blood flow increase to her pelvic region, what you'll find is a woman who's highly responsive, and who will have an orgasm much more easily.

If your jaw feels like it will fall off during oral sex with your partner and she still doesn't seem any closer to getting off, don't be afraid to bring in a toy to help you both out. It can be your secret weapon and will do a lot of the heavy lifting for you.

Using a toy in conjunction with your tongue and fingers can give her that little extra vibration that she needs to reach climax from oral. Seriously, think of how much less work your tongue has to do.

Chapter 8

Oral Sex

Giving a woman the true sexual pleasure that she CRAVES is NOT easy…

But in this chapter, I'll show you exactly how you can make it not only EASY but effortless.

I'm going to show you how to eat a girl so that you almost guarantee she has an orgasm.

I'm going to show you how to use your tongue to make a woman addicted to you.

Eating pussy is an art form – and it's something every guy should learn how to do if he wants to give his partner the ultimate gift.

Things To Do To Increase Her Pleasure

1. The Art Of Foreplay & Arousal

Getting your woman in the right frame of mind is one of the most crucial aspects of being able to give her an orgasm.

Women are emotional creatures, and it's literally impossible to give her an orgasm while she remains in a logical frame of mind (like when she's just finished work or is stressed out).

It is your duty and responsibility to get her relaxed, and turn her on so that she forgets about the stresses and worries of life. Foreplay is literally the art of taking a woman's mind from a logical state to a physical/emotional state.

REMEMBER, when it comes to arousal, logic is the enemy.

No woman has ever had an orgasm while doing algebra. Yet guys often tell me the only times their girlfriends have had orgasms is during makeup sex after an argument when emotions are running wild.

Your only goal in foreplay is to help her get into this emotional state where she can let go.

Getting "turned on" is about turning on the emotional/physical side of her mind and body.

And unlike men, women take much longer to get in the mood. Maybe you can get an erection and get ready for sex within 10 seconds, for women it could take half an hour or more.

This is when the sexual energy and arousal build up.

2. Teasing & Anticipation

Teasing and foreplay are where the power of the orgasm comes from. Imagine you have a huge bucket at the top of a ladder. The bucket holds water, but first, you need to fill up the bucket with water.

Your aim with the bucket is to make the biggest and most dramatic explosion possible when you finally decide to push the bucket of water off the ladder.

You could just put a little bit of water in the bucket and then push it off. But the explosion of water wouldn't be very big.

You could spend more time filling up the bucket and when you finally pushed the bucket off the ladder the explosion was huge.

The water is like female sexual energy. It needs time and foreplay to build up, but the longer you take to build up her energy, the bigger the orgasm explosion will be at the end.

3. Using A Blindfold To Increase Anticipation

One of the best ways to increase anticipation and excitement is to use props.

Because women can also be very self-conscious about sex, and especially about when they get their vagina licked out, a blindfold can be a great way to make her feel less self-conscious, and instead just enjoy the sensations.

Using a blindfold on her also has the extra effect of reducing one of her senses. When her sight is switched off her perception of touch will massively increase.

She will feel the sensations and stimulation from her pussy so much more.

It's also slightly scary wearing a blindfold. You will have complete control over her (which women love) and her sense of excitement and anticipation will increase.

4. Using Handcuffs/Belt/Tie To Make It Exciting

You can take her level of excitement and kink further by handcuffing her to the bed. You can either use prop handcuffs, for a more spontaneous feel, use your belt or a tie to tie her hands to the bed.

This, in combination with the blindfold and what I'm about to teach you, is the beginning of what will be one of the most exciting, powerful, sensual, and loving orgasms she will ever have.

No other guy will be able to compare to the orgasm you will give her if you follow these instructions carefully.

The Basic Techniques Of How To Eat Her Pussy Out

There are different ways to stimulate her pussy with your mouth. Each technique has its own advantages and sensations, so you'll want to use all methods at different stages of arousal.

You should also study her reactions to see which method she likes the most. Some women have very sensitive vaginas, they prefer the lighter methods.

Some women need a stronger sensation to have an orgasm, so you will need to start with methods 1 and 2 before going on to the rest.

Don't go straight to her vagina. Start by kissing her body and then work your way down. Tease her. Make every single nerve in her body come alive with sexual tension.

1. Blowing

Blowing on her pussy is a great form of arousal, foreplay, and teasing. The light, subtle sensation will begin to create sexual energy and tension (which gets released in an orgasm).

The blowing is very light, it teases and tickles her. It draws her attention and focus to the subtle sensations she feels in her pussy. This is exactly what you want. You want her in a state of hypersensitivity. Every nerve in her vagina will start tingling with sensations.

This is setting the stage for the other methods that will eventually tip her over the edge and into a body-trembling orgasm.

2. Licking

Licking is next. You can now start to use your tongue in light motions across her sensitive parts.

It's important to make your movements light and unpredictable to start with. You still want to tease her. You still want her to be waiting in anticipation (as her sexual energy continues to build).

Keep her guessing about when and how you will lick her next.

As her level of sexual arousal continues to rise, now you can begin to really start licking her out (and most importantly her clit).

The up and down motion, softly across her clit is usually the best option.

You should vary your strokes. From slow and soft to fast and hard. Always look for her reactions so you can see or hear what she likes best.

3. Kissing

Kissing her cooch is a great way to show how much you care about her. You shouldn't kiss her vagina for too long though, but your kissing should be mixed in with the other methods.

4. Sucking

Sucking is the next stage of pleasure and most women LOVE having their pussy sucked. Now you can start using your whole mouth to stimulate not just her clit, but the rest of her too.

As her arousal levels climb higher and higher she'll soon be ready for orgasm but you should continue building more and more.

Increase the speed and intensity of the sucking.

Always remember to tease and go two steps forward, one step back. Suck on her female bits for a while, then step back and kiss, lick and blow before carrying on.

5. Motorboating And Humming

Motorboating is the final method that you'll use. It is perhaps the most powerful. Here's how to do it...

Rest your lips gently around her pussy. Have your lips so they are just lightly touching and then blow out so that your lips vibrate back and forth.

This is called motorboating and sends vibrations down through her pussy. These act like shockwaves that can trigger an orgasm to take place.

Many women claim this is one of their favorite sensations.

You can alter the speed, power, and frequency of the vibrations by holding your lips tighter, or blowing harder.

Don't go crazy though.

With the motorboating method, you'll want to hold your lips over her clit and the opening to her vagina, although you can move it around and see where provides the best stimulation.

Humming is similar to motorboating but instead of actually letting your lips move, you simply rest your mouth against her vagina and hum softly.

This sends vibrations directly into her pussy that are extremely pleasurable.

For the best results, go back and forth between the methods. Mix it up and keep her guessing.

However, when you feel like she is very close to orgasm, then stick to the method that got her there and don't change it too much.

6. Put Your Finger In Her Mouth

This is a great little trick that can really drive a woman wild and can be a great way to learn exactly how your girlfriend or wife likes to have her pussy eaten.

As you continue to eat her out, take your thumb or index finger and slowly insert it into her mouth. Tell her that you want her to lick and suck on it exactly how she wants it on her female parts.

As she begins to lick and suck on your finger, copy that motion exactly onto her pussy. She will know what she likes and she will show you.

Copy her motions as she licks, sucks, massages and swirls your finger.

This is a neat trick to learn how your partner likes it. But don't use it too often. Women like the man to take control, and they like to relax as you do the work.

7. Put 1 Or 2 Fingers Inside Her

Eating her out with your mouth is one thing, but now you need to add another sensation to the mix.

This will involve inserting a finger or two into her so that you can stimulate her g-spot at the same time as her clit.

As you can imagine, stimulating her g-spot and her clit at the same time will give her twice the amount of pleasure and the 'simultaneous orgasm' that will happen as a result is extremely powerful and intense for her.

8. Insert 1 Or 2 Fingers In Her Bum

Slipping a finger in her puss isn't the only way you can give her even more pleasure.

You can massage her ass using your fingers – something a lot of women find intensely pleasurable and exciting – and it's also possible to give them anal orgasms.

You will need to use lubrication for this though – it is absolutely essential.

I also recommend using a condom. Put your two fingers inside a condom and take a large dollop of lube onto the fingers.

As you continue to eat her out slowly tease her ass. As she relaxes, begin inserting your two fingers (with a condom on and plenty of lube) slowly into her ass.

Be gentle and slow and make sure she stays relaxed.

The sensation of having her clit stimulated by your tongue – plus the sensation of having her bum massaged with your finger up her bum will be unique, exciting, and extremely pleasurable.

Or Use A Butt Plug Instead,some women love this sensation so much, but since you only have two hands you may need to remove your fingers at some point.

In this case, you can use a butt plug to give her a similar sensation while you continue to use both your hands in other ways.

9. Using A Vibrator To Guarantee Her Orgasms

Using a vibrator can be a sneaky trick to give her even more pleasure as the vibrations move through her body almost forcing her to have an orgasm.

Place the vibrator gently onto the top of your girl's pussy, just above the clit.

Do this very slowly at first. Tease her.

She will love it.

Women love a man who takes control and shows experience in the bedroom, so don't worry about using a vibrator on her.

It will show that you are thoughtful and experienced and you know how to please her sexually.

With the vibrator pressed against the top of her vagina, begin eating her out again – follow the instructions before.

Move the vibrator closer to her clit, as you continue to eat her out.

The double sensation of the vibration plus the movement of your tongue on her clit will drive her absolutely wild.

Do this right and she will have orgasm after orgasm – she won't be able to control herself.

She will beg you for more.

Now, as you rest the vibrator on her clit, and you continue to massage her labia with your mouth, take your other hand.

10. Using the lube (and a condom if necessary) begin to tickle her bum.
Slowly and gently insert one or two fingers into her bum, as you continue

to eat her out and with the vibrator held in place with your other hand.

This is the ultimate stimulation for a women. Some women even find the huge amounts of pleasure unbearable.

Her body will tremble and shake when you do this.

When you lick her out you should also have a feel for her state of arousal.

If you feel like she's about to have an orgasm, slightly slow down the pace and bring her back from the edge of climax. Doing this a few times will allow her to get into a higher and higher state of arousal before she finally climaxes.

And when she finally does cum with your tongue on her clit it will be one of the most intense orgasms she's ever had.

11. Oral Choke

A personal favorite of mine is the 'oral choke' as we call it.

With her on her back and you eating her out, extend one arm up and lightly grip around her neck.

This is a test to see if she responds positively.

If you get the feeling she likes being choked while you go down on her, you can continue and potentially tighten your grip.

Some women find the sensation of being choked (lovingly) enjoyable. It can be an effective (and novel) way to heighten the sensation of your mouth on her clit.

12. Listen to What She's Not Saying

A woman will very rarely tell you exactly what she wants. That's just not sexy for her to have to tell you.

But…

She will give you clues about what she wants most.

This is super important because, at the end of the day, not all women are the same. And they respond differently to different things.

What you'll want to do it try a few different techniques, and let her body do the speaking for her.

If she moans like crazy when you do one particular movement across her clit – DON'T STOP.

If you find the perfect rhythm, keep going at the same pace and don't change it up.

One of the biggest reasons women give for not being able to orgasm with a guy is that just before she orgasms she'll start moaning louder and louder, and this will cause the guy to change his movement or rhythm, which then causes the girl to stop moving towards her climax and preventing her orgasm.

Become a master and listening to what her body is telling you, so she doesn't have to say a word.

Become good at this, and your woman will be amazed that you 'just know what to do.'

You'll be able to read her like a book. No one else she's ever been with was able to do that.

Chapter 9

Anal Sex

Anal sex is any sexual activity that involves the anus. It does not always mean penetration with a penis. People can use sex toys, fingers, or a tongue. People of all sexual orientations and gender identities can have anal sex.

If you're curious about anal sex, you're far from alone. It may seem taboo, but behind closed doors, it turns out that more than 1 in 3 women ages 19 to 44 have tried anal sex at least once. That said, it's probably not a regular Saturday night thing. But a few things are clear: Before you try it, it's worth taking time to discuss what to know, what to avoid, and how to prepare for anal sex to make the experience amazing.

Things you need to know before you have anal sex

1. It shouldn't hurt

It may feel like an odd sensation, but done correctly, anal sex should not be painful. Unlike the vagina, the anus doesn't create its own lubrication during arousal. Try silicone-based lube; it's thicker and won't dry out the way water-based lubes can.

2. It won't "stretch you out."

Some people worry that anal sex will lead to incontinence, which isn't the case. The anus will stretch to accommodate a penis or sex toy that enters (much like it will stretch to allow a bowel movement to exit) and then will bounce back to normal.

3. It may cause an orgasm.

For some women, anal sex feels good. The anus has a rich nerve supply, which can make things feel very intense and, for some women, result in an orgasm. If she does not have an orgasm from anal sex, though, there's no reason to beat yourself up. Most women are able to achieve orgasm through clitoral stimulation, but far fewer can reach the big O through vaginal or anal sex.

4. Start slowly.

The first time you have anal sex, try it out after she's already climaxed, her body will already be relaxed and more receptive to this type of stimulation. Or you could take a shower together, and gently massage the area with a soapy finger. Experimenting in the tub or shower can also make you feel "clean," a common concern among first-timers.

5. Communicate!

Before your clothes are off, talk it out with your partner. And consider having a safe word—a code word that has nothing to do with sex (like "hockey") that brings everything to a halt, fast. This can be a smart strategy in any new sexual situation. Your partner may not be able to tell if you're making moans of pleasure or pain, so having a code word in place can make you both confident you're on the same page during the act.

6. Use condoms.

Even if you're in a monogamous relationship, condoms are a good idea when it comes to anal sex. Why? For one, they reduce friction to provide a smoother entry. Second, since anal tissue is fragile and susceptible to microscopic tears, having anal sex without a condom could cause the bacteria already in your anal canal to enter your bloodstream—not good. And use a separate condom for each sex act (like if you're going from vaginal sex to anal sex). Just be sure not to use an oil-based lube with a condom, since the oil could degrade the latex and cause the condom to break.

7. Try a toy.

Toys can be a great way to explore anal play. Make sure you find a toy suited for anal sex that has a base that flares out. Unlike the vaginal canal, which is closed, the anal canal is open and a toy could get stuck in your body. Trying a small anal plug can get your body used to the sensation of fullness and let you determine whether or not it's pleasurable.

How To Go About Having Anal Sex

If you're both open to anal sex, start in the spoon position, both lying on your sides, with you behind her. Using lots of lube, slowly and gently stimulate the area with your finger as you kiss her neck and whisper sweet, sexy things.

When you're both stimulated, try entering her slowly but not deeply, then let her control the depth. Never go too fast or deep without warming her up to the idea first. If you or she can also stimulate her clitoris with a vibrator, that can help with her arousal.

Done right, anal sex doesn't have to hurt. Start slow. Work up to it. Communicate.There is no set time for how long sex should last. It can vary greatly, depending on preference and other factors, such as what a person considers sex to be.

Not into it? Don't do it.

Although plenty of women find it pleasurable, it's not an essential to cross off your sex bucket list. Sex is supposed to be fun, and if the idea doesn't turn you on, it's totally fine to stick to your repertoire of what works.

Conclusion

Women and Sex are a huge part of my life and therefore — I take a massive interest in FEMALE SEXUALITY. In fact, I teach men how to SEXUALLY SATISFY their women..

Does Your Woman Scream Your Name When Having Sex With You? If No Make It Happen Tonight.
   You are not a real man if you have never made a woman reach orgasm, she can never be satisfied if you don't last long in bed.

You might be wondering if it is even possible for women to reach orgasms during sex. Well, naturally, they can. And, each time a woman reaches her climax, she gives out hints as to when she is about to do so by moaning in a wild manner, becoming incoherent and moving around like crazy.

After reaching their climax, women then reach a calm and deep place, making them act kittenish around you due to the sexual content that they have just experienced.

If women never seem to act this way with you after having sex, then that would mean that you have never been able to give women proper orgasms.

So, that's my challenge to all you men out there who really want to see your wives or girlfriends transform into sexually charged, super lusty vixens. Use your fingers, your tongue, a toy, whatever it takes to get her there. Give her an orgasm, then have sex — and then give her another orgasm after.

One orgasm is all it takes to turn a quiet woman into a ravenous, aggressive, hot-for-you sex fiend. Follow my advice and you just may see a side of your partner you've never seen before.

If you enjoyed this book, please take a few moments to write a review of it.

www.ingramcontent.com/pod-product-compliance
Lightning Source LLC
Chambersburg PA
CBHW060210260726
48658CB00005BA/1975